Unmasking Kidney Disease: Your Path to Lifelong Health

By

LAURA WARREN, M.D

Table of Contents

Introduction

Kidney disease, often lurking in the shadows of our health concerns, is a formidable adversary that affects millions worldwide. These vital organs, nestled deep within our bodies, play a crucial role in filtering waste and excess fluids from our blood, maintaining a delicate balance that sustains life.

However, when kidney function falters, it can give rise to a silent, yet potentially devastating condition known as kidney disease. Unbeknownst to many, its early stages often show no noticeable symptoms, earning it the moniker "the silent killer." In "Unmasking Kidney Disease: Your Path to Lifelong Health," we embark on a journey to unravel the mysteries surrounding this condition, arming you with knowledge and guidance to protect and enhance your kidney health, ensuring a path to lifelong wellness.

Throughout this book, we will explore the intricacies of kidney function, delve into the causes and risk factors of kidney disease, discuss early warning signs, diagnosis, and the array of treatment options available. We will also provide strategies for maintaining optimal kidney health, empowering you to take control of your well-being and unmask the hidden threat of kidney disease.

Chapter 1

The Hidden Threat - Understanding Kidney Disease

In this opening chapter, we embark on a journey to uncover the enigma of kidney disease, a condition often underestimated due to its silent progression. Kidneys, two small bean-shaped organs, play a vital role in maintaining our overall health, and understanding their function is key to comprehending the threat of kidney disease.

Exploring Kidney Function

- Kidneys are the body's natural filtration system, responsible for removing waste, excess fluids, and electrolytes from the bloodstream.

- They help regulate blood pressure, produce essential hormones, and maintain proper fluid and electrolyte balance.

The Silent Onset

The silent onset of kidney disease refers to the early stages of the condition when it often progresses without noticeable or alarming symptoms. This makes kidney disease challenging to detect until it reaches more advanced stages.

Some Common Reasons Why Kidney Dosease May Have a Silent Onset

1. Lack of Pain Receptors: Kidneys themselves do not have many pain receptors, so even if there is damage, it may not cause pain or discomfort.

2. Gradual Progression: Kidney disease typically develops slowly over time, allowing the body to compensate for reduced kidney function. Symptoms become noticeable as kidney function declines significantly.

3. Non-specific Symptoms: In early stages, symptoms that do occur, such as fatigue, mild changes in urine output, or slight fluid retention, are often non-specific and can be attributed to other factors or conditions.

4. Normal Blood Tests: Routine blood tests may not reveal kidney problems until kidney function is significantly impaired. Serum creatinine levels, for example, may remain within the normal range until later stages of kidney disease.

5. Asymptomatic Conditions: Some underlying causes of kidney disease, like high blood pressure or diabetes, may also be asymptomatic or have mild symptoms, which can mask the development of kidney disease.

Due to these factors, regular check-ups and screenings, especially for individuals with risk factors such as diabetes, hypertension, or a family history of kidney disease, are essential for early detection.

Detecting kidney disease in its silent onset stages allows for timely intervention and management to slow its progression and reduce the risk of complications. Many individuals are unaware of its presence until it reaches an advanced state, making early detection crucial.

Risk Factors and Prevalence

Kidney disease can result from various risk factors, both genetic and lifestyle-related. Here's a discussion of some of the key factors that predispose individuals to kidney disease:

1. Diabetes (Diabetic Nephropathy):
   - Diabetes, especially when poorly controlled, is a leading cause of kidney disease.
   - High blood sugar levels over time can damage the blood vessels in the kidneys, reducing their ability to filter waste and excess fluids.

2. Hypertension (High Blood Pressure):
   - High blood pressure is another major risk factor for kidney disease.
   - Elevated blood pressure can strain the small blood vessels in the kidneys, causing damage and reducing their efficiency in filtering the blood.

3. Family History:
   - A family history of kidney disease or a genetic predisposition can increase an individual's risk.
   - Some kidney conditions, such as polycystic kidney disease (PKD), can be hereditary.

4. Age and Gender:
   - Age is a risk factor, with kidney disease being more common in older individuals.
   - Men are generally at a slightly higher risk than women for developing kidney disease.

5. Lifestyle Factors:
   - Smoking: Smoking is associated with an increased risk of kidney disease. It can damage blood vessels and reduce blood flow to the kidneys.
   - Poor Diet: A diet high in salt, saturated fats, and processed foods can contribute to hypertension and obesity, increasing the risk of kidney disease.
   - Obesity: Excess weight can lead to diabetes and hypertension, both of which are risk factors for kidney disease.

6. Medications and Toxins:

- Certain medications, especially non-prescription pain relievers (NSAIDs), when used excessively, can harm the kidneys.
- Exposure to environmental toxins or heavy metals can also pose a risk.

7. Autoimmune Conditions:
   - Some autoimmune diseases, such as lupus and vasculitis, can cause inflammation in the kidneys, leading to kidney damage.

8. Urinary Tract Issues:
   - Conditions that obstruct the urinary tract, like kidney stones or an enlarged prostate, can increase the risk of kidney disease.

9. Infections:
   - Severe or recurrent kidney infections can lead to scarring and kidney damage over time.

10. Cardiovascular Disease:
   - Heart disease and kidney disease often go hand in hand. The presence of one condition can exacerbate the other.

Awareness of these risk factors is essential for early detection and prevention of kidney disease. Managing underlying conditions, adopting a healthy lifestyle, and regular medical check-ups can help reduce the risk and ensure better kidney health.

The increasing prevalence of kidney disease on a global scale is a significant health concern, underscoring the urgent need for awareness and prevention measures. Here are key points highlighting this growing issue:

1. Epidemic Proportions: Kidney disease has reached epidemic proportions worldwide. It is estimated that hundreds of millions of people are affected by kidney disease, making it a global public health challenge.

2. Rising Incidence: The incidence of kidney disease is steadily rising across all age groups and demographics. This increase is attributed to various factors, including an aging population, unhealthy lifestyles, and the global rise in conditions like diabetes and hypertension.

3. Global Healthcare Burden: Kidney disease places a substantial burden on healthcare systems. The cost of treating kidney disease, especially in its advanced stages, is substantial, affecting both individuals and societies.

4. Limited Awareness: One of the concerning aspects of kidney disease is the lack of awareness among the general population. Due to its often asymptomatic early stages, many individuals remain undiagnosed until the disease has progressed significantly.

5. Preventable Causes: A significant portion of kidney disease cases is preventable. Lifestyle factors such as poor diet, lack of exercise, and smoking contribute to the development of conditions like diabetes and hypertension, which are leading causes of kidney disease.

6. Importance of Early Detection: Early detection of kidney disease is crucial for effective management and slowing its progression. Routine check-ups, blood pressure monitoring, and kidney function tests can aid in early diagnosis.

7. Prevention Through Education: Raising awareness about the risk factors and prevention of kidney disease is vital. Educating individuals about maintaining a healthy lifestyle, managing chronic conditions, and recognizing the importance of

regular screenings can help mitigate the rising prevalence.

8. Promoting Kidney Health: Encouraging kidney-healthy behaviors, such as consuming a balanced diet, staying hydrated, and avoiding smoking and excessive alcohol consumption, can significantly reduce the risk of kidney disease.

9. Global Initiatives: Various international organizations and health agencies are working to address the growing prevalence of kidney disease. They emphasize the importance of preventive measures, early intervention, and improved access to healthcare services.

In conclusion, the increasing prevalence of kidney disease is a global health crisis that necessitates immediate attention. Heightened awareness, education, and proactive measures for prevention are essential to curb this rising trend and improve kidney health on a global scale. By taking action at both individual and community levels, we can make strides in reducing the impact of kidney disease and improving the well-being of millions of people worldwide.

Stages of Kidney Diseases

Kidney disease is typically classified into stages based on the estimated Glomerular Filtration Rate (eGFR), a measure of kidney function. The stages help healthcare providers assess the severity of kidney damage and determine appropriate treatment strategies.

1. Stage 1 - Kidney Damage with Normal or High eGFR ($\geq$90 ml/min):
   - In this early stage, there is evidence of kidney damage, such as protein in the urine (albuminuria), but the eGFR is normal or even high.
   - Kidney function is still relatively preserved, and individuals may not experience noticeable symptoms.

2. Stage 2 - Kidney Damage with Mildly Reduced eGFR (60-89 ml/min):
   - Kidney damage continues, but there is a slight decrease in eGFR.
   - Individuals in this stage may still not experience significant symptoms, and kidney function is generally adequate for daily activities.

3. Stage 3 - Moderate Reduction in eGFR (30-59 ml/min):
 - In this stage, kidney function is moderately reduced.
 - Some symptoms may start to appear, such as fatigue, mild swelling, and changes in urine output.
 - Management and lifestyle changes become increasingly important to slow the progression of kidney disease.

4. Stage 4 - Severe Reduction in eGFR (15-29 ml/min):
 - Kidney function is significantly impaired in Stage 4.
 - Symptoms can become more pronounced, including swelling, fatigue, increased blood pressure, and changes in urine patterns.
 - Preparation for renal replacement therapy (dialysis or transplant) may be necessary in advanced cases.

5. Stage 5 - End-Stage Renal Disease (ESRD) (<15 ml/min or dialysis):
 - This is the most severe stage of kidney disease, where kidney function is critically impaired.

- Individuals often experience severe symptoms such as extreme fatigue, fluid retention, nausea, and electrolyte imbalances.
- Treatment options include dialysis or kidney transplantation, as the kidneys can no longer adequately filter waste and excess fluids from the bloodstream.

It's important to note that kidney disease is a progressive condition, but its progression can often be slowed or managed with appropriate medical care, lifestyle changes, and early intervention. Regular monitoring and timely treatment are crucial, especially as the disease advances through these stages. Early detection and management in the earlier stages (1-3) can significantly improve outcomes and quality of life for individuals with kidney disease.

The stages of kidney disease progress in a manner where kidney function gradually declines, and symptoms become more pronounced as kidney function deteriorates. The correlation between stages, kidney function, and symptoms highlights the importance of early detection and intervention in the earlier stages to slow the progression of the disease and improve the overall quality of life for individuals with kidney disease.

Complications of Kidney Disease

1. Cardiovascular Complications: Kidney disease significantly increases the risk of cardiovascular problems. These include high blood pressure, heart disease, heart attacks, and strokes. Kidney disease can lead to the buildup of fluid and sodium in the body, putting additional strain on the heart and blood vessels.

2. Anemia: Damaged kidneys may produce less of the hormone erythropoietin, leading to anemia. Anemia results in a reduced number of red blood cells, causing fatigue, weakness, and pale skin.

3. Mineral and Bone Disorders: Kidneys play a vital role in regulating calcium and phosphorus levels in the body. When kidney function declines, these minerals can become imbalanced, leading to bone diseases like osteoporosis and vascular calcification.

4. Electrolyte Imbalances: Kidney disease can disrupt the balance of electrolytes in the body, such as potassium and sodium. Severe imbalances can affect muscle function, nerve function, and even lead to cardiac arrhythmias.

5. Fluid Retention and Edema: As kidney function declines, the body may retain excess fluid, leading to swelling, particularly in the ankles, legs, and around the eyes.

6. Metabolic Acidosis: Kidneys help maintain the body's acid-base balance. When they don't function properly, it can result in metabolic acidosis, leading to muscle and bone problems and potentially affecting vital organ function.

7. Uremia: Uremia is a syndrome in which waste products normally filtered by the kidneys accumulate in the bloodstream. This condition can lead to nausea, vomiting, itching, and mental confusion.

8. Neuropathy: Kidney disease can cause nerve damage, leading to peripheral neuropathy.

Symptoms may include tingling, numbness, and
pain in the hands and feet.

Beyond Kidney Disease

1. Impact on Quality of Life: Kidney disease can
have a profound impact on an individual's quality of
life. The need for dialysis or transplantation can be
emotionally and physically challenging.

2. Financial Burden: Treating kidney disease,
especially in its advanced stages, can be costly.
Expenses related to dialysis, medications, and
hospitalizations can place a significant financial
burden on individuals and their families.

3. Risk of Infection: Kidney disease can weaken the
immune system, making individuals more
susceptible to infections.

4. Psychological and Emotional Effects: Coping
with a chronic illness like kidney disease can lead to
stress, anxiety, depression, and a decreased overall
sense of well-being.

5. Life Expectancy: The progression of kidney disease can impact life expectancy. Timely diagnosis and management can improve outcomes and extend life.

In summary, kidney disease is not limited to its impact on the kidneys alone; it can have far-reaching consequences for an individual's overall health, well-being, and quality of life. Early detection, management, and lifestyle modifications are critical in mitigating these complications and improving outcomes for those affected by kidney disease.

- Kidney disease doesn't affect just the kidneys; it can lead to various complications, including cardiovascular problems, anemia, and bone disease.
- Emphasize thThe ripple effect of kidney disease on overall health is profound and multifaceted, touching various aspects of a person's well-being.

Here, we emphasize how kidney disease can impact not only the kidneys but also other systems and aspects of health:

1. Cardiovascular System: Kidney disease significantly increases the risk of cardiovascular problems, including high blood pressure, heart disease, heart attacks, and strokes. The kidneys and the cardiovascular system are closely intertwined, and the strain placed on the heart and blood vessels can lead to a cascading effect of health issues.

2. Metabolic Health: Kidneys play a pivotal role in regulating various metabolic processes. When they are compromised, it can disrupt the balance of electrolytes, leading to issues like high potassium levels (hyperkalemia) and metabolic acidosis. These imbalances can affect muscle function, bone health, and overall metabolic stability.

3. Bone Health: Kidney disease can lead to mineral and bone disorders, including osteoporosis and vascular calcification. This not only weakens the bones but also increases the risk of fractures and complications related to bone health.

4. Hematological System: Anemia is a common complication of kidney disease due to reduced production of erythropoietin. Anemia can result in fatigue, weakness, and reduced oxygen delivery to tissues, affecting overall vitality.

5. Immune Function: Kidney disease can weaken the immune system, making individuals more susceptible to infections and hindering the body's ability to fight off illnesses effectively.

6. Neurological Health: Nerve damage, known as peripheral neuropathy, can occur as a result of kidney disease, leading to symptoms such as tingling, numbness, and pain in the extremities. This can affect mobility and overall neurological well-being.

7. Psychological and Emotional Health: Coping with a chronic illness like kidney disease can take a toll on one's psychological and emotional health. Stress, anxiety, depression, and a diminished sense of well-being are common in individuals dealing with the challenges of kidney disease.

8. Nutritional Status: Kidney disease often necessitates dietary restrictions to manage electrolyte imbalances and fluid retention. These restrictions can impact an individual's nutritional status and dietary enjoyment, affecting overall health and quality of life.

9. Endocrine System: Kidneys are involved in regulating hormone levels in the body. When kidney function declines, it can disrupt hormone balance, leading to various endocrine issues.

10. Quality of Life: The physical, emotional, and financial burdens of kidney disease can have a profound effect on an individual's overall quality of life. It can limit activities, impact relationships, and create a sense of uncertainty about the future.

In conclusion, kidney disease is not isolated to the kidneys; it has a far-reaching and interconnected impact on multiple systems and aspects of an individual's health. Recognizing and addressing the ripple effect of kidney disease is crucial for comprehensive care, emphasizing the importance of early detection, management, and holistic support to improve the overall health and well-being of those affected.

The ripple Effect of Kidney Disease on Overall Health

The ripple effect of kidney disease on overall health is profound and multifaceted, touching various aspects of a person's well-being. Here, we emphasize how kidney disease can impact not only the kidneys but also other systems and aspects of health:

1. Cardiovascular System: Kidney disease significantly increases the risk of cardiovascular problems, including high blood pressure, heart disease, heart attacks, and strokes. The kidneys and the cardiovascular system are closely intertwined, and the strain placed on the heart and blood vessels can lead to a cascading effect of health issues.

2. Metabolic Health: Kidneys play a pivotal role in regulating various metabolic processes. When they are compromised, it can disrupt the balance of electrolytes, leading to issues like high potassium levels (hyperkalemia) and metabolic acidosis. These

imbalances can affect muscle function, bone health, and overall metabolic stability.

3. Bone Health: Kidney disease can lead to mineral and bone disorders, including osteoporosis and vascular calcification. This not only weakens the bones but also increases the risk of fractures and complications related to bone health.

4. Hematological System: Anemia is a common complication of kidney disease due to reduced production of erythropoietin. Anemia can result in fatigue, weakness, and reduced oxygen delivery to tissues, affecting overall vitality.

5. Immune Function: Kidney disease can weaken the immune system, making individuals more susceptible to infections and hindering the body's ability to fight off illnesses effectively.

6. Neurological Health: Nerve damage, known as peripheral neuropathy, can occur as a result of kidney disease, leading to symptoms such as tingling, numbness, and pain in the extremities. This can affect mobility and overall neurological well-being.

7. Psychological and Emotional Health: Coping with a chronic illness like kidney disease can take a toll on one's psychological and emotional health. Stress, anxiety, depression, and a diminished sense of well-being are common in individuals dealing with the challenges of kidney disease.

8. Nutritional Status: Kidney disease often necessitates dietary restrictions to manage electrolyte imbalances and fluid retention. These restrictions can impact an individual's nutritional status and dietary enjoyment, affecting overall health and quality of life.

9. Endocrine System: Kidneys are involved in regulating hormone levels in the body. When kidney function declines, it can disrupt hormone balance, leading to various endocrine issues.

10. Quality of Life: The physical, emotional, and financial burdens of kidney disease can have a profound effect on an individual's overall quality of life. It can limit activities, impact relationships, and create a sense of uncertainty about the future.

In conclusion, kidney disease is not isolated to the kidneys; it has a far-reaching and interconnected impact on multiple systems and aspects of an individual's health. Recognizing and addressing the ripple effect of kidney disease is crucial for comprehensive care, emphasizing the importance of early detection, management, and holistic support to improve the overall health and well-being of those affected.

The Role of Early Detection

- The importance of routine screenings for the early detection of kidney disease cannot be overstated, especially for individuals at risk. Here are compelling reasons why routine screenings are vital:

1. Silent Progression: Kidney disease often advances silently in its early stages, showing no noticeable symptoms. Routine screenings can detect the disease before it reaches an advanced, symptomatic state, making early intervention possible.

2. Prevent Progression: Early detection allows healthcare providers to implement measures to slow or halt the progression of kidney disease. This can

significantly improve long-term outcomes and quality of life.

3. Reduce Complications: Identifying kidney disease early can help prevent or manage complications. Timely treatment and lifestyle modifications can reduce the risk of cardiovascular problems, anemia, bone disease, and other associated issues.

4. Preserve Kidney Function: Early intervention can help preserve kidney function and delay or even prevent the need for dialysis or transplantation in advanced stages of the disease.

5. Manage Underlying Conditions: Routine screenings may identify underlying conditions like diabetes and hypertension, which are leading causes of kidney disease. Managing these conditions effectively can reduce the risk of kidney disease development.

6. Cost-Effective: Detecting kidney disease early is cost-effective. It can save individuals and healthcare systems significant expenses associated with treating advanced kidney disease and its complications.

7. Empowerment: Knowing your kidney health status empowers you to make informed decisions about your lifestyle, diet, and healthcare. It allows for proactive steps to maintain or improve kidney function.

8. Individuals at Risk: Individuals with risk factors such as diabetes, hypertension, a family history of kidney disease, or a history of kidney infections should prioritize regular screenings. Early detection is especially critical for this high-risk group.

9. Public Health Impact: Widespread routine screenings can have a positive public health impact by reducing the overall burden of kidney disease, leading to healthier communities.

10. Advancements in Treatment: Early diagnosis opens doors to various treatment options, including medications, lifestyle changes, and dietary modifications. Staying informed about your kidney health ensures you can benefit from advancements in medical care.

In conclusion, routine screenings for kidney disease, especially for individuals at risk, are an essential component of proactive healthcare. Early detection not only improves individual outcomes but also has far-reaching implications for public health. By prioritizing kidney health and seeking regular screenings, individuals can take control of their well-being and work towards preventing or managing kidney disease in its early and more manageable stages.

The significance of simple tests like serum creatinine and eGFR in assessing kidney function

Serum creatinine and estimated Glomerular Filtration Rate (eGFR) are fundamental tests used to assess kidney function. They provide critical information about how well the kidneys are working. Here's a discussion on the significance of these tests:

1. Serum Creatinine:
   - What it Measures: Serum creatinine is a waste product generated by muscle metabolism. It is filtered out of the blood by the kidneys and excreted in the urine.

- Significance: Elevated serum creatinine levels indicate that the kidneys may not be effectively clearing this waste product from the bloodstream. This suggests impaired kidney function.

- Early Warning: Serum creatinine levels may begin to rise when kidney function is already moderately impaired, making it a valuable early warning sign.

2. eGFR (Estimated Glomerular Filtration Rate):

- What it Measures: eGFR is a calculated estimate of the kidneys' filtration rate. It assesses how much blood the glomeruli (tiny filtering units in the kidneys) can filter per minute.

- Significance: eGFR provides a more precise assessment of kidney function compared to serum creatinine alone. It is a better indicator of overall kidney health.

- Staging Kidney Disease: eGFR values are used to categorize the stages of kidney disease. Values below 60 ml/min/1.73m² indicate decreased kidney function.

- Monitoring: eGFR values can be tracked over time to monitor changes in kidney function, allowing for early detection of declining function.

The Significance of Combining Both Tests

- Comprehensive Assessment: Together, serum creatinine and eGFR offer a comprehensive assessment of kidney function. While serum creatinine alone can detect impaired function, eGFR provides a more accurate estimate and helps categorize the stage of kidney disease.

- Early Detection: The combination of these tests is crucial for early detection of kidney disease. A decrease in eGFR or an increase in serum creatinine can indicate kidney problems even before symptoms appear.

- Monitoring: Regularly tracking both serum creatinine and eGFR values allows healthcare providers to monitor kidney function over time. Any significant changes can prompt timely intervention or adjustments to treatment plans.

- Treatment Decisions: eGFR values play a pivotal role in treatment decisions, especially in advanced stages of kidney disease. They help determine the need for interventions like dietary changes, medications, or dialysis.

- Risk Assessment: For individuals at risk of kidney disease due to conditions like diabetes or hypertension, these tests are essential for ongoing risk assessment and early intervention.

In conclusion, serum creatinine and eGFR are key tests in assessing kidney function. Serum creatinine provides a basic indicator of kidney health, while eGFR offers a more precise estimate and helps stage kidney disease. Regular monitoring of these parameters is essential for early detection, intervention, and effective management of kidney disease, contributing to better overall health and quality of life.

Chapter 2

Unveiling the Culprits - Causes and Risk Factors

This chapter delves into the root causes and risk factors that underlies the development of kidney disease. Kidney disease does not occur in isolation; it is often a consequence of various contributing factors.

Understanding the Causes

1. Diabetes (Diabetic Nephropathy):
   - Diabetes, particularly Type 1 and Type 2, is a leading cause of kidney disease.
   - High blood sugar levels can damage the blood vessels in the kidneys, impairing their filtration function.

2. Hypertension (High Blood Pressure):
   - High blood pressure is another primary cause of kidney disease.
   - Elevated blood pressure can strain the small blood vessels in the kidneys, leading to damage over time.

3. Genetics and Family History:
   - Genetic predisposition plays a role in certain kidney diseases, such as polycystic kidney disease (PKD) and Alport syndrome.
   - A family history of kidney disease can increase an individual's risk.

Lifestyle and Behavioral Factors

4. Smoking:
   - Smoking is linked to kidney disease, as it can damage blood vessels and reduce blood flow to the kidneys.
   - Smoking cessation is a crucial step in reducing this risk.

5. Poor Diet:

- Diets high in salt, saturated fats, and processed foods can contribute to hypertension and obesity, both risk factors for kidney disease.
- A balanced diet with reduced sodium intake is recommended.

6. Obesity:
- Excess weight is associated with an increased risk of kidney disease, as it can lead to diabetes and hypertension.
- Weight management is crucial for kidney health.

7. Lack of Physical Activity:
- A sedentary lifestyle is linked to obesity and increased risk of hypertension and diabetes, all of which are risk factors for kidney disease.
- Regular physical activity can mitigate these risks.

8. Urinary Tract Issues:
- Conditions that obstruct the urinary tract, such as kidney stones or an enlarged prostate, can increase the risk of kidney disease.

9. Infections:
- Recurrent or severe kidney infections can lead to kidney damage over time.

10. Medications and Toxins:

 - Certain medications, especially non-prescription pain relievers (NSAIDs), can harm the kidneys when used excessively.

 - Exposure to environmental toxins or heavy metals can also pose a risk.

In essence, this chapter serves as a critical eye-opener to the causes and risk factors contributing to kidney disease. By emphasizing the role of modifiable risk factors, genetic factors, and the importance of early detection and prevention strategies, this chapter equips readers with the knowledge and motivation to take proactive steps in safeguarding their kidney health.

Chapter 3

Early Warning Signs - Recognizing Kidney Disease Symptoms

This chapter focuses on the critical importance of recognizing the early warning signs and symptoms of kidney disease. It aims to empower individuals to be proactive in seeking medical attention if they experience any of these symptoms.

Recognizing the Symptoms

1. Changes in Urination:
   - Frequent Urination: An increased need to urinate, especially at night, may indicate kidney dysfunction.
   - Decreased Urination: Conversely, reduced urine output or oliguria can signal impaired kidney function.

2. Blood in Urine (Hematuria):
   - The presence of blood in the urine, even in small amounts, should never be ignored. It can be a sign of kidney injury or underlying kidney disease.

3. Swelling (Edema):
   - Swelling, particularly in the ankles, legs, feet, or around the eyes, can result from fluid retention due to impaired kidney filtration.

4. Fatigue and Weakness:
   - Persistent fatigue and weakness can be early signs of anemia, a common complication of kidney disease.

5. Shortness of Breath:
   - Difficulty breathing or shortness of breath, especially during physical activity, may be linked to fluid buildup in the lungs caused by kidney-related heart issues.

6. High Blood Pressure:
   - Unexplained or sudden high blood pressure, especially in previously normotensive individuals, can be a warning sign of kidney problems.

7. Metallic Taste in Mouth and Ammonia Breath:
   - The buildup of waste products in the blood can lead to unusual tastes and breath odors, often described as metallic or ammonia-like.

8. Nausea and Vomiting:
   - Persistent nausea and vomiting, especially accompanied by a loss of appetite, can result from the accumulation of waste products in the bloodstream.

Bone and Muscle Problems

9. Muscle Cramps and Twitching:
   - Muscle cramps and twitching can occur due to electrolyte imbalances resulting from kidney dysfunction.

10. Bone Pain and Fractures:
   - Kidney disease can lead to mineral and bone disorders, causing bone pain and an increased risk of fractures.

Neurological and Cognitive Changes

11. Difficulty Concentrating and Mental Fog:
   - Cognitive changes, including difficulty concentrating and mental fog, can be associated with kidney disease, particularly in advanced stages.

However, chapter 3 highlights the significance of recognizing early warning signs and symptoms of kidney disease. It encourages readers to be vigilant about changes in their health and seek timely medical evaluation when they encounter these symptoms.

Empowering individuals to be vigilant about these symptoms and seek prompt medical evaluation can lead to early detection and intervention, ultimately improving kidney health and overall quality of life. Early recognition of these signs is the first step toward better kidney care and long-term well-being.

Chapter 4

Diagnosis and Beyond - Navigating the Kidney Disease Journey

Diagnosis and Beyond - Navigating the Kidney Disease Journey is a chapter that addresses the comprehensive process of managing kidney disease, from initial diagnosis to the ongoing journey of care. Let's explain its meaning in full:

- This chapter serves as a guide for individuals diagnosed with kidney disease, their families, and healthcare providers.
- It acknowledges that receiving a diagnosis is just the beginning of a lifelong journey with kidney disease and aims to provide a roadmap for understanding, managing, and thriving despite the challenges.

Understanding the Diagnosis of Kidney Disease

Understanding the diagnosis of kidney disease is a crucial first step in managing this condition effectively. Let's explore this aspect in detail:

1. Medical Evaluation: The diagnosis often begins with a medical evaluation, including a review of your medical history and risk factors. Your healthcare provider will ask about symptoms, family history, and any chronic conditions like diabetes or hypertension.

2. Laboratory Tests:
   - Serum Creatinine: One of the primary diagnostic tests is the measurement of serum creatinine levels in your blood. Elevated levels may suggest reduced kidney function.

   - eGFR (Estimated Glomerular Filtration Rate): eGFR is calculated based on your serum creatinine levels and is used to estimate your kidney function. A low eGFR indicates potential kidney problems.

- Urinalysis: A urine test can detect abnormalities like proteinuria (excess protein in the urine) and hematuria (blood in the urine), which can be signs of kidney disease.

- Imaging: Imaging tests like ultrasounds, CT scans, or MRIs may be used to visualize the kidneys and identify structural issues.

3. Staging Kidney Disease: Once a diagnosis is confirmed, kidney disease is typically categorized into stages based on eGFR values. This staging helps determine the severity of the condition and guides treatment decisions.

4. Identifying Underlying Causes: It's essential to determine the underlying causes of kidney disease, which can range from diabetes and hypertension to genetic factors or urinary tract issues. Identifying the cause informs treatment strategies.

5. Patient Education: A crucial part of understanding the diagnosis involves patient education. Healthcare providers should explain the implications of the diagnosis, the stage of kidney disease, and the importance of proactive management.

6. Potential Complications: Patients should be informed about potential complications associated with kidney disease, such as anemia, cardiovascular problems, and bone disorders. Early awareness can lead to timely interventions.

7. Treatment Options: Patients need to understand the various treatment options available, including medications, dietary modifications, and lifestyle changes. In advanced stages, discussions about dialysis and transplantation may be necessary.

8. Monitoring: Patients should be aware of the need for ongoing monitoring of kidney function, blood pressure, and other relevant parameters. Regular check-ups help track disease progression and treatment effectiveness.

9. Proactive Self-Care: Understanding the diagnosis empowers individuals to actively participate in their care. Patients can take steps to manage their condition through proper medication management, dietary choices, and lifestyle adjustments.

10. Emotional Support: Acknowledging the emotional impact of a kidney disease diagnosis is crucial. Patients should be encouraged to seek emotional support from loved ones, support groups, or mental health professionals to cope with the challenges.

In summary, understanding the diagnosis of kidney disease involves a comprehensive evaluation, diagnostic tests, patient education, and awareness of treatment options and potential complications. This knowledge is the foundation for individuals to actively manage their condition and work collaboratively with healthcare providers to improve kidney health and overall well-being.

Emphasizing the importance of recognizing kidney disease early and understanding the significance of specific tests like serum creatinine and eGFR cannot be overstated.

Here's why early recognition and these tests are so crucial:

1. Early Detection Saves Lives: Kidney disease often progresses silently, without noticeable

symptoms in its early stages. By the time symptoms become evident, the disease may have advanced significantly. Early detection through tests like serum creatinine and eGFR allows for timely intervention, potentially preventing further damage and complications.

2. Slowing Disease Progression: Kidney disease is often progressive, but its rate of progression can vary. Early detection provides an opportunity to implement measures that can slow or even halt the progression of the disease. This can significantly improve long-term outcomes and quality of life.

3. Preventing Complications: Kidney disease is associated with a range of complications, including cardiovascular problems, anemia, bone disorders, and more. Identifying kidney disease early can lead to interventions that reduce the risk of these complications or manage them effectively when they occur.

4. Preserving Kidney Function: Early intervention can help preserve kidney function. While kidney disease may not be curable, its progression can be managed. Slowing the decline in kidney function is

critical in avoiding the need for dialysis or transplantation in advanced stages.

5. Optimizing Treatment: Understanding kidney disease early allows healthcare providers to tailor treatment plans to the individual's specific needs. Medications, dietary recommendations, and lifestyle changes can be initiated promptly to achieve the best possible outcomes.

6. Preventing Acute Kidney Injury: Early detection of kidney disease can also help prevent acute kidney injury (AKI), a sudden decline in kidney function that can be life-threatening. Recognizing and managing kidney disease reduces the risk of AKI triggers.

7. Monitoring Progress: Kidney function can fluctuate, and the disease may progress differently in each individual. Regular monitoring, initiated early, helps healthcare providers track changes in kidney function over time, allowing for timely adjustments to treatment plans.

8. Education and Empowerment: Early diagnosis provides an opportunity for patient education.

Individuals can learn about the causes of kidney disease, the role of specific tests, and the importance of lifestyle modifications. This knowledge empowers them to take an active role in their healthcare.

9. Reducing Healthcare Costs: Detecting kidney disease early is cost-effective. It can save individuals and healthcare systems significant expenses associated with treating advanced kidney disease and its complications.

In conclusion, recognizing kidney disease early and understanding the significance of tests like serum creatinine and eGFR are pivotal in improving outcomes and quality of life for individuals affected by this condition. Early detection is a lifeline that offers the best chance for effective management, reduced complications, and a brighter future for kidney health.

Acceptance and Emotional Support

Acceptance and emotional support play an essential role in navigating the journey of kidney disease. Here's why they are crucial:

Acceptance

1. Acknowledging the Diagnosis: Acceptance begins with acknowledging the kidney disease diagnosis. It's a critical step in coming to terms with the condition and its potential impact on one's life.

2. Empowerment: Acceptance empowers individuals to take control of their health. It shifts the focus from denial or fear to proactive steps towards managing the condition effectively.

3. Reducing Stress: Acceptance can reduce stress and anxiety associated with the diagnosis. It allows individuals to face the reality of their situation and seek support without the added burden of denial or avoidance.

4. Positive Mindset: Acceptance fosters a positive mindset. When individuals accept their condition, they are more likely to engage in self-care, adhere to treatment plans, and maintain a hopeful outlook.

Emotional Support

1. Family and Friends: Emotional support from family and friends is invaluable. Loved ones can provide a strong foundation of understanding, empathy, and encouragement during challenging times.

2. Support Groups: Kidney disease support groups offer a sense of belonging and understanding. Interacting with others who share similar experiences can provide emotional validation and practical advice.

3. Mental Health Professionals: Sometimes, the emotional impact of kidney disease may require professional assistance. Mental health professionals can offer strategies to cope with stress, anxiety, depression, or grief related to the diagnosis.

4. Education and Communication: Emotional support often comes from being well-informed about the condition. Healthcare providers should ensure that patients and their families receive clear, empathetic explanations of the diagnosis and its implications.

5. Empathy and Compassion: Healthcare providers should approach patients with empathy and compassion, recognizing the emotional challenges they may face. An understanding healthcare team can make a significant difference in the patient's experience.

6. Patient Advocacy: In some cases, patients may require advocates who can help them navigate the healthcare system, understand their treatment options, and ensure their emotional needs are met.

7. Advance Care Planning: Emotional support is essential when discussing advance care planning, including end-of-life preferences. Having these conversations with loved ones and healthcare providers can relieve emotional burdens and ensure that the patient's wishes are respected.

In conclusion, acceptance and emotional support are cornerstones of coping with kidney disease. They empower individuals to face their diagnosis with resilience, reduce emotional distress, and improve overall well-being. Recognizing the emotional toll of kidney disease and providing the necessary support can make a profound difference in the patient's journey.

Treatment Options for Kidney Disease

1. Medications:
   - Blood Pressure Medications: Controlling high blood pressure is crucial to slowing kidney disease progression. Medications like ACE inhibitors and ARBs are commonly prescribed.

   - Diuretics: These drugs help the body eliminate excess fluid and reduce swelling (edema).

   - Medications for Anemia: Erythropoietin-stimulating agents (ESAs) and iron supplements may be prescribed to manage anemia associated with kidney disease.

- Phosphate Binders: In advanced stages, medications may be necessary to control high phosphorus levels in the blood.

2. Dietary Modifications:
   - A renal diet, often guided by a registered dietitian, can help manage electrolyte imbalances and reduce stress on the kidneys. It may involve restricting sodium, potassium, phosphorus, and protein intake.

3. Lifestyle Changes:
   - Lifestyle modifications such as regular physical activity, smoking cessation, and maintaining a healthy weight can positively impact kidney health.

4. Control of Underlying Conditions:
   - Managing underlying conditions like diabetes and hypertension is essential. Keeping blood sugar and blood pressure levels within target ranges helps protect kidney function.

5. Dialysis:
   - Dialysis is a life-saving treatment for individuals with advanced kidney disease. There are two primary types:

- Hemodialysis: A machine filters the blood outside the body and returns it after waste removal.

- Peritoneal Dialysis: A special solution is introduced into the abdominal cavity, where it absorbs waste and excess fluid. It is then drained out.

6. Kidney Transplantation:
- Kidney transplantation is considered the best treatment option for end-stage kidney disease. A healthy kidney from a living or deceased donor replaces the failing kidney. Transplants offer improved quality of life and longevity compared to dialysis.

7. Vascular Access Surgery:
- For individuals on hemodialysis, vascular access surgery may be required to create a suitable vein for dialysis access. This can involve arteriovenous (AV) fistulas, AV grafts, or central venous catheters.

8. Advanced Therapies:
- In some cases, advanced therapies such as immunosuppressive drugs or experimental

treatments may be considered, particularly for specific kidney diseases or transplant patients.

9. Monitoring and Preventive Care:
   - Regular monitoring of kidney function, blood pressure, and other relevant parameters is essential to track the progression of kidney disease and adjust treatment plans as needed.
   - Preventive care, including vaccinations and infection management, is crucial for individuals with compromised kidney function.

It's important to note that the choice of treatment depends on the stage and cause of kidney disease, individual health factors, and patient preferences. Treatment plans are often individualized and may evolve over time as the condition progresses. Effective kidney disease management requires close collaboration between healthcare providers and patients to determine the most suitable treatment approach for each case.

Diet and Nutrition for Kidney Disease

Diet and nutrition play a pivotal role in managing kidney disease effectively. Here's a comprehensive overview of the dietary considerations for individuals with kidney disease

1. Control of Protein Intake:
   - In early stages of kidney disease, a moderate reduction in protein intake may be recommended. This helps reduce the burden on the kidneys, as protein breakdown can produce waste products.

   - High-quality protein sources like lean meats, poultry, fish, and eggs are preferred to minimize waste production.

2. Sodium (Salt) Restriction:
   - Limiting sodium intake is crucial, as excess sodium can lead to fluid retention and high blood pressure, both of which can worsen kidney disease.

   - Foods high in sodium, such as processed foods, canned soups, and restaurant/fast food, should be minimized.

3. Potassium Management:
   - Individuals with kidney disease may need to monitor potassium intake, as high levels can disrupt heart rhythm.

   - Foods rich in potassium, such as bananas, oranges, and potatoes, may be limited or portion-controlled.

4. Phosphorus Control:
   - Elevated phosphorus levels can occur in advanced stages of kidney disease, leading to bone problems and other complications.

   - A dietitian may recommend limiting phosphorus-rich foods, such as dairy products, nuts, and certain processed foods.

5. Fluid Restriction:
   - In advanced stages of kidney disease, fluid intake may need to be restricted to avoid fluid overload, which can lead to edema and high blood pressure.

   - Individualized fluid allowances are determined by healthcare providers.

6. Calcium and Vitamin D:

  - Kidney disease can affect calcium and vitamin D metabolism. Calcium supplements and vitamin D may be prescribed as needed to maintain bone health.

7. Healthy Fats:

  - Healthy fats from sources like avocados, nuts, and olive oil should be included in the diet to provide essential nutrients and calories.

8. Calorie Management:

  - Weight management is crucial. For those with kidney disease and obesity, calorie intake may need to be controlled to achieve or maintain a healthy weight.

9. Monitoring Nutrient Levels:

  - Regular blood tests are essential to monitor nutrient levels, including potassium, phosphorus, and calcium. Dietary adjustments are made based on these results.

10. Consulting a Renal Dietitian:

  - A registered dietitian with expertise in renal nutrition can provide personalized dietary guidance, taking into account the individual's stage of kidney disease, nutritional needs, and preferences.

11. Balanced Diet:
   - A balanced diet with a variety of fruits, vegetables, whole grains, lean proteins, and limited processed foods is recommended for overall health.

12. Meal Planning:
   - Creating a meal plan that aligns with dietary restrictions and preferences can help individuals with kidney disease adhere to their dietary recommendations.

13. Fluid Intake Education:
   - Education on measuring and tracking fluid intake is essential, especially for those with fluid restrictions. It helps individuals make informed choices about beverages and foods with high water content.

14. Medication Management:
   - Some dietary restrictions may be influenced by medications prescribed to manage kidney disease and related conditions. It's important to follow medication instructions closely.

In summary, diet and nutrition are integral components of kidney disease management. A well-planned and individualized diet can help slow the progression of kidney disease, manage complications, and improve overall well-being. Consulting a registered dietitian with expertise in renal nutrition is strongly recommended to ensure that dietary choices align with individual health needs and treatment goals.

Importance of Regular Monitoring

Regular monitoring is a crucial aspect of managing kidney disease effectively. Here's why it's so important and what it involves:

1. Disease Progression Tracking: Kidney disease can progress slowly, and its rate of progression varies among individuals. Regular monitoring allows healthcare providers to track changes in kidney function over time, helping them understand how the disease is advancing.

2. Treatment Adjustment: Monitoring provides insights into the effectiveness of treatments and

interventions. If kidney disease progresses or if complications arise, healthcare providers can adjust medications, dietary plans, and other aspects of care accordingly.

3. Complication Prevention: Regular check-ups can help prevent or detect complications associated with kidney disease, such as high blood pressure, anemia, bone disorders, and cardiovascular problems. Early intervention can mitigate these risks.

4. Medication Management: Kidney disease often requires medications to manage related conditions like hypertension and anemia. Monitoring ensures that medications are dosed correctly and that their effects are assessed regularly.

5. Nutritional Guidance: For individuals following a renal diet, monitoring helps dietitians assess nutritional status, adjust dietary plans, and manage nutrient imbalances like potassium and phosphorus levels.

6. Fluid Management: For those with fluid restrictions, monitoring fluid intake is crucial to prevent fluid overload, edema, and high blood

pressure. Individuals learn to make informed choices about their fluid intake based on monitoring results.

Components of Regular Monitoring

1. Blood Tests: Blood tests are commonly used to monitor kidney function. These tests include serum creatinine, eGFR, and blood urea nitrogen (BUN). They provide insights into waste product levels in the blood and how well the kidneys are filtering.

2. Urine Tests: Urinalysis can detect abnormalities such as proteinuria (excess protein in the urine) or hematuria (blood in the urine). Changes in urine composition can signal kidney problems.

3. Blood Pressure Monitoring: Regular blood pressure measurements are essential, as hypertension is a common complication of kidney disease. Blood pressure control is critical in slowing disease progression.

4. Electrolyte Levels: Periodic checks of electrolyte levels (e.g., potassium, sodium, calcium, phosphorus) help manage nutrient imbalances, which can affect heart and bone health.

5. Imaging: Imaging tests such as ultrasounds, CT scans, or MRIs may be performed to visualize the kidneys and assess structural issues.

6. Medication Review: Healthcare providers review medication regimens to ensure that medications are being taken correctly and that any side effects are addressed.

7. Nutritional Assessments: For individuals on a renal diet, dietitians regularly assess nutritional status and make necessary adjustments to dietary plans.

8. Review of Symptoms: Patients are encouraged to communicate any new or worsening symptoms or side effects during monitoring visits.

Frequency of Monitoring

The frequency of monitoring varies depending on the individual's stage of kidney disease and overall health. Typically, individuals with more advanced kidney disease or those at higher risk of complications require more frequent monitoring, often every few months. Those in earlier stages may have less frequent check-ups, but monitoring remains a lifelong commitment for individuals with kidney disease.

In conclusion, regular monitoring is a cornerstone of kidney disease management. It allows healthcare providers to assess disease progression, adjust treatment plans, and prevent complications effectively. Patients are encouraged to actively participate in their monitoring process and communicate openly with their healthcare team to ensure the best possible kidney health outcomes.

Chapter 5

Lifelong Wellness - Strategies for Kidney Health and Prevention

Maintaining lifelong kidney health is crucial. Here are some strategies for kidney health and prevention:

1. Hydration: Stay well-hydrated by drinking enough water throughout the day to help your kidneys filter waste effectively.

2. Balanced Diet: Consume a balanced diet rich in fruits, vegetables, whole grains, and lean proteins while limiting sodium, sugar, and processed foods.

3. Manage Blood Pressure: Keep your blood pressure in check, as high blood pressure can harm your kidneys. Monitor it regularly and follow your doctor's recommendations.

4. Control Diabetes: If you have diabetes, manage your blood sugar levels through medication, diet, and exercise to prevent kidney damage.

5. Healthy Weight: Maintain a healthy weight to reduce the risk of kidney disease and related conditions.

6. Limit Alcohol and Avoid Smoking: Excessive alcohol consumption and smoking can harm your kidneys. It's best to avoid them or use them in moderation.

7. Regular Exercise: Engage in regular physical activity to help maintain a healthy weight and overall well-being.

8. Medication Management: Take medications as prescribed by your healthcare provider and be aware of any potential kidney-related side effects.

9. Avoid Overuse of Painkillers: Non-prescription pain relievers like NSAIDs can harm your kidneys if overused. Use them sparingly and follow the recommended dosage.

10. Get Regular Check-ups: Visit your healthcare provider for regular check-ups and kidney function tests, especially if you have risk factors like diabetes or high blood pressure.

11. Manage Stress: Chronic stress can negatively impact your overall health, including kidney function. Practice stress-reduction techniques like meditation and deep breathing.

12. Limit Phosphorus and Potassium: If you have kidney disease, manage your phosphorus and potassium intake as advised by your healthcare provider.

13. Monitor Protein Intake: If you have kidney issues, your doctor may recommend adjusting your protein intake. Follow their guidance.

14. Stay Informed: Educate yourself about kidney health and potential risk factors to make informed choices.

15. Limit Salt Intake: Reducing your sodium (salt) intake helps control blood pressure and minimizes

the strain on your kidneys. Aim for less than 2,300 milligrams of sodium per day.

16. Control Protein Intake: If you have kidney disease, your doctor may recommend moderating your protein consumption. High protein diets can strain the kidneys, so consult with a healthcare provider or a registered dietitian for personalized guidance.

17. Monitor Blood Sugar: For individuals with diabetes, tight blood sugar control is vital to prevent kidney damage. Regularly monitor your blood glucose levels and adhere to your diabetes management plan.

18. Avoid Excessive Caffeine: Too much caffeine can potentially increase blood pressure, so moderate your coffee and tea intake.

19. Maintain a Healthy Blood Cholesterol Level: High cholesterol levels can lead to kidney damage. Follow a heart-healthy diet, exercise regularly, and take prescribed medications if needed.

20. Stay Active: Regular physical activity can help control weight, lower blood pressure, and reduce the risk of kidney disease. Aim for at least 150 minutes of moderate-intensity exercise per week.

21. Limit Alcohol Consumption: Excessive alcohol can disrupt kidney function, so drink in moderation, if at all. The recommended limit is up to one drink per day for women and up to two drinks per day for men.

22. Stay Informed About Medications: Some medications, like certain antibiotics and pain relievers, can be harmful to the kidneys if misused or overused. Always follow your doctor's instructions and inform them of all medications you're taking.

23. Manage High Blood Pressure: If you have hypertension, work closely with your healthcare provider to manage it effectively. This often involves medication and lifestyle changes.

24. Know Your Family History: Understanding your family's medical history can help identify genetic factors that may increase your risk of kidney

disease. Share this information with your healthcare provider.

25. Avoid Overuse of Herbal Supplements: Some herbal remedies and supplements may affect kidney function. Consult with a healthcare professional before using any new supplements or herbs.

26. Get Vaccinated: Certain infections, like hepatitis B and C, can lead to kidney problems. Ensure you're up to date on vaccinations and take precautions to avoid exposure.

27. Stay Hydrated, But Don't Overdo It: While it's important to stay hydrated, excessive water intake can strain the kidneys. Aim for about 8-10 cups of water daily, or as advised by your doctor.

28. Seek Prompt Treatment: If you experience symptoms like persistent fatigue, changes in urination, blood in urine, or swelling, don't hesitate to seek medical attention. Early detection and treatment can prevent kidney disease from progressing.

Remember, kidney health is an essential part of overall well-being, and preventive measures are key to lifelong wellness. Always consult with a healthcare professional for personalized advice and guidance.

Conclusion

In conclusion, kidney health is of paramount importance for overall well-being and longevity. Kidney disease can have far-reaching consequences, but with proactive measures and a commitment to a healthy lifestyle, it can often be prevented or managed effectively. Here are key takeaways:

Lifestyle Matters: Kidney health is closely tied to your overall lifestyle choices. A diet rich in fruits, vegetables, whole grains, and lean proteins not only benefits your kidneys but also supports your entire body's health. Regular physical activity not only helps maintain a healthy weight but also promotes good circulation and blood pressure, reducing the risk of kidney disease. Avoiding smoking and limiting alcohol intake are additional steps you can take to protect your kidneys from harm.

Regular Monitoring: Routine check-ups are your first line of defense against kidney disease. These appointments provide an opportunity for healthcare providers to assess your kidney function and detect any early signs of trouble. For those with underlying health conditions like diabetes or high blood pressure, frequent monitoring is particularly crucial to ensure timely intervention and prevent kidney damage from progressing.

Medication Adherence: Medications prescribed to manage conditions like hypertension or diabetes are effective tools in preventing kidney complications. Adhering to your medication regimen as prescribed by your healthcare provider is vital. It's not just about managing the condition itself but also safeguarding your kidney health for the long term.

Hydration and Diet: Kidneys rely on proper hydration to filter waste and toxins from your blood. Drinking an adequate amount of water daily supports their function. Additionally, maintaining a diet low in sodium (salt), sugar, and processed foods can significantly reduce the strain on your kidneys. These dietary choices promote not only kidney health but also heart health and overall well-being.

Consult a Healthcare Provider: The guidance of a healthcare provider is invaluable when it comes to kidney health. They can offer personalized advice, monitor your condition, and recommend specific lifestyle changes or treatments tailored to your unique needs. If you're at risk or have kidney disease, consulting with a nephrologist (kidney specialist) can provide specialized care.

Stay Informed: Knowledge is a powerful tool for protecting your kidney health. Being aware of risk factors, symptoms of kidney problems, and preventive measures empowers you to make informed decisions. Stay curious, ask questions, and seek reliable sources of information to stay informed about your kidney health.

By prioritizing these aspects of kidney health throughout your life, you not only reduce the risk of kidney disease but also contribute to your overall well-being. Taking proactive steps to care for your kidneys is an investment in a healthier and longer life.